The Autism Guide to Sayings and Slang:
Contains Crass Concepts and Coarse Language

By Tristan Johnson

TRISTAN JOHNSON

ISBN-13: 978-1519715838
ISBN-10: 1519715838

TABLE OF CONTENTS

INTRODUCTION

This is no literary tome.

I simply had that "deer in the headlights" look when people used slang and sayings. For years, I mean a lot of years, I had heard the saying, "busier than a one-handed paper hanger," and I had no clue what it meant. I pictured a clothing hanger hanging in a closet with paper attached to it with a clothes pin. But, I was puzzled about how a hand came in to play.

I never asked because I didn't want to be laughed at or told I'm stupid—both of which I painfully remember from being in school. I'm 49, so you would think I have gotten over it, but some of the mean kids in school have grown up to be hyper-critical adults—"assholes" for short.

And, since I'm on the autism spectrum, it is hard to know who is a good and safe person and who isn't. Whether they are good or not, I can feel pretty clueless in a conversation due to the sheer number of sayings and slang people use. I mean, WTF?—an acronym for "what the fuck?"

While my children were growing up, I remained blissfully oblivious since I really didn't know anybody. I usually had one friend and that's it. I have noticed over the years that most of my friends have been the quiet types.

Except my friend David. He was an outgoing, hyper-talkative type, but the biggest thing is that he was very accepting of others, unless they screwed him around, of course, then he was hell on wheels, so any warm-bodied human had better get out of his way.

I never had to worry about his wrath because I'm so nice. Really. I am born to be mild. (It's a play on words from "born to be wild," which is commonly applied to Harley motorcycle riders.)

Dave taught me some sayings and slang, but for most of my adult years, I didn't even realize that I had difficulty with them until I got older. It came out during work meetings and interpersonal interactions. I remember being at a meeting and the guy talking said, "It'll all bubble up." What the hell is that?

My children became teenagers so the slang flew hot and fast. I could talk teen-speak with the kids and their friends because they taught me. The difference in this situation is that I was "Dad," so I wasn't expected to know, so no judgment.

The big change came when I started dating my wife. She has spent her work life in engineering, and she currently works for Big Technology Company that works with Other Big Companies, and boy do they talk slang.

They use acronyms I know, such as SQL being "structured query language," but that dratted "busier than a one-armed paper hanger" stumped me. Corporate America is mired in sayings and slang, and she uses them like the best of them.

But my wife and I were quickly relationship bound, so I felt safe enough to ask her what the hell she was talking about. After we moved in together, I started asking her the meaning of sayings, and since she likes watching cable news, I was constantly asking because they seem to use sayings and slang as often as possible.

So, just for fun, I started writing down sayings on a steno pad one summer. I got most of them from my wife, TV news channel pundits, and the oh-so-serious writers at TIME magazine. Newspaper headlines are so lame because they write things like, "Auto Dealer Drives a Hard Bargain."

When it comes to this not being a literary tome, I'll explain why.

As I had mentioned, I'm 49, so I'm not hip on what nine-year-olds are saying, but I do remember "gnarly" from the 80s. I'm a white, suburban, middle-income, independent-voting man, so I may not necessarily know slang or sayings from other sociographic groups.

Please be easy on me when you write or talk about this book; attack the content, not me.

VERY IMPORTANT

If you are on the spectrum, don't use these sayings and slang unless you are sure of the context to use them in.

But, how will you know which sayings are okay and which aren't? How do you know what context to use them in? You will have to ask your parent, a friend or sibling who knows about sayings, or a skills worker who helps you on appropriate social interaction.

See this guide as a way to understand what other people are meaning, not for you to use the sayings and slang yourself. That is the safest route so you don't unwittingly offend others even though you mean no harm.

Learn them as you go. For example, if you go to visit at your aunt's house, don't say, "What the fuck, I haven't seen you in a long time." "Fuck" is generally a no-no.

However this one is good: "Wow, he's had a tough go of it, but he has risen to the occasion." That is praise, and people will like that you said it.

HOW TO FIND THINGS IN THIS BOOK

If you are reading an electronic version of this book, you have it made. All you have to do is look up something by key word. Not so easy if you have the print version. I will do my best to keep to the first word as how to alphabetize the sayings, but it doesn't always work well.

For example, I will not have all sayings that begin with "the" listed in the "T" section. Another example would be, "all washed up," which would be in the "W" section for "washed" as the keyword.

I will also not alphabetize a saying by "he" or "she." Most of the sayings can use the "he," "she," or "they" interchangeably.

0

One fell swoop
Done all at once

3 sheets to the wind
Really drunk on booze.

Third wheel
When a couple is together, having a third person in the awkward situation is uncomfortable.

10 feet under
Dead, as buried in the ground.

40 winks
A night's sleep

69
When two people are facing the other's feet and performing oral sex on each other.

86ed
Kicked out from somewhere.

800-pound gorilla in the room
The gorilla is not an animal, rather, it is the name of an idea or information or feeling known by two or more people involved in the situation, but don't talk about it. The gorilla is ignored even though everyone knows it's there.
Can also be substituted with "elephant in the room."

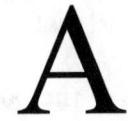

Above board
Honest.
Forthcoming.
Open.

Don't know him from Adam
Don't know him at all.

Have your a-game on
Doing your best.

Against the grain
Like rubbing fur backwards.
Going against the flow.

Airhead
Not very smart.

Air your dirty laundry
Tell about the inside, not-so-good details about your life.

All bark and no bite
Someone who talks a lot but doesn't do any action.
Someone who is harmless.

All that jazz
All that stuff.

All the power to ya
Go ahead.
Do it.

An eye for an eye
Retribution.
Evening the score.

Ants in your pants
Antsy.

Bad apple
Bad person.
A person with negative energy or behavior that brings other more virtuous people down to his low level.

Half assed
Not doing something properly or completely, usually because he doesn't care to do it right.

Ass over tea kettle
Fall.

Aunt Flo
A funny euphemism for when a woman is menstruating. Often used as "Aunt Flo has come to visit," meaning that a woman's period has started.

At the end of her rope
Reached the limit.

Axe to grind
An issue or problem with a person or situation.

TRISTAN JOHNSON

B

Back against the wall
No way out.
Stuck.
Tough situation.
Nowhere to go or hide.

Back Stabber
Someone you had trusted and was nice to you, does or says something mean to you or says mean things about you to other people.
A person you had trusted with your secrets turns around and tells them to others without you knowing.

Back to the drawing board
Starting over.

Bad
Good, as in, "that is so bad."

(He's) bad news
Troublesome person.

Bad ass
A bad person, usually a man, who is intimidating because he could hurt someone or does bad things, such as breaking the law. An example would be the

stereotype of the dangerous biker—as in Harleys, not people dressed in tights driving $800 titanium bicycles.
On the fringe of cool—not that it isn't cool, but because it's SO cool, it's highly desirable or admired.

Bad egg
Bad or rotten person.

Baked
High on drugs, most often, marijuana.

Half baked
An idea that is not thought through.
An idea that has little promise.

Ball buster
Really tough problem or situation.

Balls
Testicles.

Ballsy
Gutsy.
Brave, maybe to excess.

Bananas
Crazy.

Banging her head against the wall
Extremely frustrated with a situation.
A situation is stalled after trying so hard to give it impetus.

Barking up the wrong tree
Asking or going to the wrong person.

Goes to bat for you
A person defends you or rallies others to you, possibly with a personal risk.

Beat him to the punch
Be first.

Beating around the bush
Avoiding the topic.
Being evasive.

Beats me
I don't know.

Beat the bush
Looking for something.
Trying to search something out.

Beaver
Vagina, usually referring to the hair on the vagina.

Has a bee in her bonnet
She is mad or angry or upset. This saying is more often used with women.

Been around the block (a time or two)
Experienced.
Derogatory term for someone who is sexually promiscuous.

Been fed a line
Lied to.
Deceived.

Been had
Have been taken advantage of.
Believe a person who has lied to you.

Been sold a bill of goods
Lied to.
Deceived.

Beeotch
A slangy way of saying "bitch."

Beggars can't be choosers
Someone who is asking for something for free, but wants a certain thing, or a better thing than what is offered. The person being asked will be annoyed or angry that the requestor does not want to settle for what is offered, which can result in the offer being withdrawn.

Belly-aching
Complaining
.

Beside myself (him- or her-self)
Overly something such as joy, anxiety, sorrow,
excitement, and more.
Extreme state of some emotion.

(Got the) best of her
Took advantage.

Between you and me and the light post
Secret.
Don't tell anyone.
Confidential.

Beyond the pale
Excessive.
Beyond belief.

Big-headed
Thinks too much of herself.
The mind is filled with grandiose ideas.

Big wig
Powerful person high up in the hierarchy of an
organization.

A bird in the hand is better than two in the bush
A bird in your hand is something you have. The two
in the bush you don't have, and may never have.
This means taking a chance on getting two instead of
keeping the once is foolhardy. It's for people who
don't like to take risks or people who are considered
prudent.

Birds of a feather flock together
Like things get along or hang out together.

Bite the bullet
Face the situation.
Face the pain.
Get it done.

A bitter pill to swallow
Tough task.

Bit the dust
Died

Bite me
A very rude way to say "no." It's almost as bad as "fuck off."

Bite off more than you can chew
Take something more than you can handle.

That bites
Something is unfortunate or bad.

Bite the hand that feeds him
Attack his friends who support him.
Wrongfully attacking those who are good to you.

Bleeding heart
Excessively compassionate.

Bless his heart
A polite euphemism to describe a person with less than usual intellectual capability.

Blew it
Made a mistake.

Blind ambition
So much ambition that the person sees nothing else in her path.

Blind faith
Have faith in something not yet known or achieved.

Blood on her hands
Guilty of something.
The person is responsible for something bad.

Blow him/it off
Ignore him.

Blow off some steam
Releasing tension.
Getting tension out.

Blowing smoke up my ass
Trying to convince with an untruth.
Majorly twisting the truth to try and get you to accept that twisted truth.

Blow job
Performing fellatio—sucking a man's penis.

Blow it all
Spend all your money on things that are not needed instead of being frugal and perhaps saving or investing the money.

Blue balls
Excessively sexually aroused and frustrated because there is no relief.

Whatever floats your boat
Sure, you do what you like even though it's not something I would do.

What it boils down to
After the extraneous has been stripped away, the core of the situation or idea is revealed.

(It's the) bomb
Really good.

Bombed
Drunk on alcohol.
An endeavor failed badly.

Bone
Penis.

Boner
A dumb thing to do
An erect penis.

Boondoggle
Waste of time.

Booty
Bum or butt.

Boots under your bed
Pretend you are listening to a plaintive country song.
A man will take off his cowboy boots and put them
under a woman's bed in preparation for sleeping
with her, so it means that he is having sex with her.

Born to be wild
The name of a song recorded by the band
"Steppenwolf" in the 60s. It was used on the
soundtrack for the movie, "Easy Rider," about two
bikers experiencing the counter-culture of the 70s
and the societal upheaval of the time. It became
synonymous with the biker culture.
It can also be used as a "lighter" version. For
example, I can get all dressed up like a "suburban
woman gone wild" for the evening out dancing with
hubby. I'm hardly a tough, road-hardened biker, so
the saying takes on a bit of a comical turn. This is
why I call myself "born to be mild."

Born with a silver spoon in his mouth
Born into a life of privilege.
Parents are wealthy.

Boost (booster)
Steal.

The bottom line
The absolute last that can be done
The truth about the situation that cannot be refuted or argued against.

Boys will be boys
Excusing behavior as normal or expected of a boy or man.

No-brainer
Extremely simple to understand.
Should be self-evident.
It is the way that the concept is universally known.

Brass balls
Brave.
Strong.

Break a leg
Good luck, usually before someone goes on stage to perform.

Break the ice
When two people don't know each other, conversation is started about something they both have in common like something trivial such as weather or coffee or location, which makes them feel more comfortable.

One brick short of a load
Missing some intelligence.
Not that intelligent.

Not the brightest bulb on the Christmas tree
Mentally dim as in dumb.

Bring home the bacon
Earn the money for the household

Bring it on
Heartily welcomes the activity or the challenge.

Bros before hos
Men who are loyal to their friends ahead of women.

Brown as a berry
Suntanned

Brownie points
Earning favors.
Good deeds.
Good will.

Brushing him off
Ignoring someone.

See what bubbles up
An action is undertaken, but the results are not known, so start the action and see what happens and what the result will be.

Bucko bucks
Lots of money.

The buck stops here
Taking responsibility.

Bug bear
Something that annoys people or causes problems.
Continuing source of irritation.

Bugger
Tough.
Hard.

Buggered up
Broken.

Bugger off
Tell a person to go away.
Leave.

Bug in your ear
Trying to get their attention.

Bug up your ass
Feeling like you are antsy to get doing something.
Feeling or acting in an antsy way.
Determined to pursue something.

Bullshit
Not true.
Not believable.

A bum's rush
Forcible ejection.
Hurrying someone away.

Bum rap
Falsely accused.

Bumping uglies
Having sex.

Bump on a log
Not doing anything.
Not active or involved.

Burn a mule
Go for a poo.

Burn the candle at both ends
Doing something that is hard to keep up.
Doing a combination of things that are physically and/or intellectually taxing so much so that a breakdown of the activity or the mind may ensue.
Can't keep up the activity for a long time.

Burning a hole in my pocket
In reference to money, that you feel urgency to spend it.

Burning the midnight oil
Working late.

Bury the hatchet
Make peace.

His/her business
Genitals.

Busier than a one-handed paper hanger
A person who is hanging wallpaper with one hand, so it requires constant movement to try to get the wallpaper up.

(It's a) bust
A flop.
A failure.

Bust his balls
Challenge.

Bust your bubble
Disappoint.

Busy body
A person who is overly concerned about other people's affairs and sometimes interfering in them.

Butter fingers
Awkward or clumsy.
Drops things.

Butter him up
Try to gain favor with by being excessive nice and saying sweet things.

Buzz kill
Ruining the fun.
Were happy, but another person came along who made the situation sad.
Previously excited, hyped up, then someone, the buzz kill, comes along and ruins the happy mood.

Buzz off
Go away.

By hook or by crook
One way or another.
Whatever it takes.

C

Cake walk
Easy to do.

Call a spade a spade
Tell it like it is.

Calling her out
Revealing in front of others the bad action or words that a person has taken, often seeking retribution.

Call the shots
Lead.
Make the decisions.

A come on
Being excessively nice to gain favor or achieve a purpose through someone.

Canary in the coal mine
Indicator.
Warning.

Holds a candle for you
Likes you and thinks about you.
Romantically inclined to you.

On the can
Sitting on the toilet to pee or poo.

Candy ass
A person who is weak in a derogatory, dismissive way.
A person who is not tough enough for the situation.

Can't get blood out of a stone (or turnip)
One wants something, usually money, that another person doesn't have.

Can't hold a candle to you
You are the best, the original person that others cannot emulate.
No one is better than you are.

Can't put the toothpaste back in the tube
Can't take it back.
Can't start over.

Can't teach an old dog new tricks
Difficult to change existing behavior.

Carry a torch for her
Pine for.
I love with her.
Unrequited love.

Cash cow
Source of money or funding.

The cat's ass
The best it can be.
Something is really awesome.

The cat's meow
Really good.
The best a situation or thing can be.

The cat's out of the bag
A secret you didn't want found out is now revealed.

Caught between a rock and a hard place
In a difficult situation.
At a standstill.

Caught red-handed
Caught in the act, usually of doing a crime.

Caught with his hands in the cookie jar
Caught stealing.

Caught with his pants down
Caught in an awkward situation.

Cement shoes
Made popular as a part of popular mafia culture that was purported to mean that a person who wasn't paying their protection money or who had done wrong to the mafia had their feet dried in concrete then dumped in the river to drown.

(You're) chicken
Scared to do something.

Chicken little
Excessively or easily worried.

Chicken shit
Person who is scared.

Chill (out)
Relax.

Chin up
Be happy.
Raise your spirits.

Chip on his shoulder
Viewing life as bad or unfair and views others with envy for having more than he perceived he does.

Choked
Failed under pressure.

Chop chop
Hurry up.

Chump
Someone who is used.

Circling the wagons
Becoming defensive.

Clam up
Stop talking.
Refusal to talk.

Clean as a whistle
Very clean.

Cleaned his clock
Won.
Easily won a fight.

Clear the air
Openly discuss a situation.

Clean up your act
Get one's life in order.
Stop doing illegal things.

Clocked him
Punched him really hard, often meaning that he was knocked out.

Close but no cigar
Almost.

Close to the vest
Secretive.

Clue in
Figure out.

Clueless
Doesn't know anything.

Clusterfuck
The situation is as bad and disorganized and in such array that the people dealing with it are bemoaning their situation.

Chin wagging
Talking light conversation.
Senseless talking.

Coast is clear
As in being pursued, it is safe to proceed.

Cock
Penis.

Cock-eyed
Off center.
Crooked.
Off balance.

Cold feet
Apprehensive.
Not sure.
Agreed to do something, then got really scared as the event approached, and he gets really scared and doesn't want to do it anymore.

Colder than a well digger's ass
Really chilled to the bone after being chilled for a longer time. This is how a well digger's ass is because his ass is pressed up against the wall of the well, which is cold and wet.

Cold shoulder
Ignore.

Come back to bite you
A problem that returns.

Come in from the cold
Gain insight.
Learn.
Understand.

Come out of the closet
Revealing that you are gay.

Come unglued
A situation or emotion that feels like the situation or one's world has fallen apart.

Comments from the peanut gallery
Insignificant people not related to the cause that have no place commenting on it.

Come clean
Tell the truth when a person had been lying.
Do a situation rightly when he had been doing it deceitfully.

Come hell or high water
Whatever it takes.

Come out of his shell
Open up.
Become more outgoing.
Come to Jesus meeting
Serious meeting.
Lay down the law.
Disciplinary meeting.

Coming out of the woodwork
All over the place.
Lots.

Cook the books
Create accounting that misrepresents the actual numbers to avoid being found out, which could lead to prosecution.

Cool beans
Agree.
Will do it.
Like it.

Cool your heels
Relax.
Slow down.
Wait.

Cool your jets
Relax.
Wait.

Costs an arm and a leg
Expensive.

Cougar
Older women, perhaps over 40, who date younger men.

Cover his ass
Doing or saying things that helps him to not get harmed or blamed in a situation.

Cracks me up
Makes me laugh.

Croaked
Died

Take a crack at it
Try something, usually when someone else has tried and failed.

Crash (out)
Go to sleep.

Crap
Poo.
Useless.

(Oh) crap
Darn.

(All) Crapped out
Tired.
Worn out.

Crap shoot
Random.
Unknown outcome.
Taking a chance.

Crashed out
Sleeping, often in a deep sleep from exhaustion.

(I've) created a monster
Unleashed something bigger than expected.

Crock of shit
Lies.

Cross your Ts and dot your Is
Make sure all the details are covered.
Review carefully.

Cup of joe
Coffee.

Cut and dried
Simple.
Only one answer.

Cut a rug
Dancing.

Cute as a button
Cute.
Attractive.

Cut his nose off to spite his face
Do something to hurt someone else, but it ends up hurting yourself.

Cut the crap
Stop it.
Stop lying.

Cut the mustard
Is up to the task.

Cut to the chase
Stop evading or even lying about something implied.
State in a straight-forward manner.
Get to the bare truth.

TRISTAN JOHNSON

D

Dag nabit
Darn.

Daisy chain
String of daisies tied together.
Can daisy chain elements together.
A circle of women each performing cunnilingus on another (licking a vagina) while also receiving cunnilingus. This can be with gay men or heterosexual people also.

Dangling a carrot in front of his nose
Tempting.
Enticing.
Leading.

In the dark
Have no knowledge of a situation, often by people who know, but don't want you to know.

Day late and a dollar short
Too late.

Dead in the water
The situation or endeavor is over with or never came to fruition.

Dead soldier
Empty bottle of booze.

Deep pockets
Has a lot of money.

Deer in the headlights look
Look confused.
Stuck.

Dense
Not very intelligent.

Desk jockey
Someone who works at a white collar job at a desk or in a cubicle.

Devil's advocate
Take another point of view.
Taking a negative opposing view.

Dialed in
On track.
On task.
Focused.

Dick wagging
Bragging.
Trying to sound better than someone else.

Different breed of cat
Unusual, but not in a bad way. Meant more that the person is unusual, interesting, and pleasing.

Dilly dallying
Not on task.
Slow.
Not acting with a sense of urgency.

A dime a dozen
There is plenty of something worth no special notice or acclaim.

Ding dong
Dummy.

Dip your wick
Sexual intercourse.

Dippy
Dumb.

Dirt bag
Not a good person.
Uncouth person.

Dirt poor
So poor that they are reduced to eating dirt since food is so scarce.

Going the distance
Taking an idea or endeavor as far as you can take it.
Doing something not done previously or does it
better than others.

Doesn't have a pot to piss in
Really poor.

Doesn't pass the sniff test
It stinks.
Not truthful.
Easily exposed as false.

Don't buy it
Doesn't believe it.

Don't give a fuck/patoot/hoot/shit/rat's ass
Don't care.

Don't give a fat flying fuck
Don't care emphatically.

Doesn't say boo to him
Doesn't say anything.
Extremely shy.

Do one over on him
Deceived him.
Did better than him.

(Such a) dog
Ugly.
A tough problem with no easy answer.
A man who is a slut.

(It's a) dog eat dog world
Only the strongest survive.
The world is difficult to deal with.
You must compete to get ahead.

(In the) dog house
In trouble.

Dogging it
Acting slowly.

A dog's breakfast
Confused mess.
A muddle.

Dog tired
Really tired or worn out.

Going to the dogs
Becoming destroyed or wearing down into ruin
Becoming less than so the endeavor is becoming
ruined.
Not as good anymore and will probably land up in
ruin.

All dolled up
All dressed up and looking good.

Done for/done in
Exhausted and can't do more.
Feel beaten.

Don't pull any punches
Tell it what the situation is.
Open and honest.9i

Don't take any shit
Stand up for yourself.

A doozie
Extreme.
Really good or really bad.

Dope
So cool, awesome, likeable.

Got the dope on
Learned the inside details of a situation.

Down in the dumps
Sad.

Dough
Money.

Doubled down
Sticking with an activity, even against the odds.
Trying again.

Down for the count
Dead.
No longer effective.
Go to sleep.

Down with
Like.

Douche (bag)
An unlikable person.

Down and dirty
Getting down to business.

Down in the dumps
Feeling lackluster.
Sad, but not necessarily having a full-blown, clinical depression.

A real downer
Something that lowers everyone's mood, as in disappointment.

Down in the dumps
Sad.

Down to the wire
At the last minute.

Down with that
Like it.
Will participate in it.

Do you hear me?
Do you understand me?

Dozey
Sleepy.
Not very smart.

Dragging your feet
Delaying.
Avoiding.

Drive me around the bend
Making me feel frustrated, angry, or disorganized by something you are doing.

Drink it up
Experience something fully.
Absorb knowledge.

(In the) driver's seat
In charge.

A drop in the bucket
Only a little bit, a miniscule bit of the entire picture.

Drop the dime on
Tell on someone.
Tattle.

Hung out to dry
People who you trusted let you down and let you take the blame for something.

Drunk out of his ass
Very, very drunk to the point of slurring speech, staggering, blacking out, and/or passing out.

(Get your) ducks in a row
Get ready for something by organizing.

(It's a) Duck walk
Easy.

Just ducky
Good.
Everything is not so good (sarcastic)

Dumb as a stump
Really stupid.

Dumped me
Doesn't want to be your girlfriend/boyfriend anymore.

Dust off
Take a project that has been left idle and start it again.

TRISTAN JOHNSON

E

Ear to the ground
Paying attention to.
Listening for.

Easy peasy
No problem because it's easy to do.

Easy as pie
Extremely easy to do.

Eat a sandwich
Said to a person who is skinny.

Eat crow
Be humbled.
Admit you are wrong.

Eat her out
Lick a woman's vagina and clitoris as a sexual method.

Eat his dust
Trying to keep up.

Eat worms
Take your punishment, sometimes self-inflicted.

Eat your heart out
One person in a favorable situation or has something favorable or desired, that person will say that to another because they perceive that they have something the other wants.

Eat your words
Being found out.
Humbled.

What's eating you?
What's the matter?
What is consuming your thoughts that it bothers and distracts and saddens you?

Eats like a bird
Eats very little and grazes all day.

There's only one way to eat an elephant—one bite at a time.
This not literally eating an elephant. The elephant stands for a concept or knowledge to understand or huge task to be undertaken that is so big that the only way to understand or accomplish it is to do one small part at a time.

Egg on his face
Embarrassed.

All your eggs in one basket
Depending on a single thing or outcome.
No alternative plan.

Elbow grease
Work hard.

Enough of that noise
Don't want to hear any more about that.

Every dog has its day
Everybody gets their turn.
Everyone gets one shot at fame or accomplishment.

Your eyes are bigger than your stomach
Taking on more than you can handle.
Taking more food than you can eat at a meal.

F

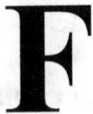

Face the music
Admit your mistake.

Fag hag
A heterosexual girl who hangs out with gay guys.

Fair to midlan
Average.
Okay.

Fair weather friends
Likes you only when things are going well with you.
Not a true friend.

Falling out
Having a disagreement.
Having a fight.

Fall on your can
Fall over.
Fall on your butt.

Family jewels
The husband's testicles

Fat
Rich.

Fat cat
Rich person.

Fat, dumb, and happy
This is a saying often used to describe ex-wives who receive an ample monthly alimony check.
Any person who doesn't work and is in a good, moneyed life situation. This saying is sometimes applied to stay-at-home mothers to partners with a good income.
A totally unambitious person living off of welfare with no ambition to do anything else.

(Dropping the) F-Bomb
The word "fuck"

Feather in your cap
An accomplishment.

Feeling blue
Sad, melancholy, though less than a debilitating depression.
Sometimes a person will say that another person is in a debilitating depression when they don't wish to say how serious the depression is.

Feeling no pain
Drunk.
Oblivious.

Feeling punky
Feeling slow, not energized, maybe coming down with a cold.

Got itchy feet
Antsy and anticipating, sometime impatiently, for something to happen, usually something anticipated that is a big event in a person's life.
Antsy and impatient to get going and go forward.

Think on your feet
In a situation, instead of knowing all that will be done ahead of time, you think and do as the situation emerges.

(Hold his) feet to the fire
Hold responsible for.

(Getting his) feet wet
Starting.
Learning.
Initial attempt.

Fell for her
Fell in love.

Fell off the wagon
Started drinking booze again when the person had been sober.
Started something again.

Fence sitter
Bisexual person.
Undecided person.

Fight tooth and nail
Fight with passion.

Fighting an uphill battle
A losing battle.
Very difficult.
Probably aren't going to win.

Go figure
Who would have thought that would happen.

Finagling
Deceiving.

Find herself
A person may not be doing something that is
congruent with her inner self. The process of
learning her inner self is finding herself and
changing her life to make her inner and outer life
congruent.

Can't put my finger on it
Don't remember but may at any moment by thinking
hard.
Can't quite figure something out, but may at any
moment.

Has her fingers in too many pies
Activities are spread too thin.
Trying to do too much.

Fire in his belly
Really energized to undertake something, and
undertakes it with zeal.

All fired up
Very excited about something.
Ready to take excited action now.

Fits the bill
Appropriate fit.

Fit to be tied
Mad.
Really mad.

Flaked out
Getting weird or unstable.
Went to sleep.

Flash in the pan
Short-lived.

Fleshed out
Filled in the details.

Flew over my head
Didn't understand.

Flip her off/the bird
Giving the "fuck you/fuck off" sign with your middle finger with the rest of the fingers closed in a fist.

Flying low
Ill.
Low energy.

Fly by night operation
An enterprise that is shady, edging close to or over the legal line.

Flying by the seat of her pants
Reckless.
Doing without thinking.
Without having a definite path.

Fly off the handle
Get angry and yell.
Quickly angered.
Inappropriately angered without knowing the details.
Leaping without looking.

On the/Fly on the straight and narrow
Honest almost to a fault.
Not versed in uncouth things and doesn't do uncouth things.
Does things legally and honestly.

(Wish I could be a) Fly on the wall
Listen in.

Foot in mouth disease
Saying stupid things.
Misspeaking.

Force his hand
Make him do something.

A fool's errand
Mistake.

For the birds
Unnecessary.
Wasteful.
Useless.

Foot loose and fancy free
Without a care.
Happy.
Free.

For Pete's sake
When someone does, or says, or hears something,
the person is not happy with the situation and feels
upset or unbelieving.

Forty winks
Sleep a night.

Fried
Become high on marijuana or another drug.

Going to get fried out there
While lying in the sun, you will get a sun burn.
Putting one's self out there, such as giving a political speech or debate, and getting verbally beaten on.

From soup to nuts
From A-Z.
Start to end.
Complete.

From the frying pan into the fire
Going from a bad situation into one that is even worse.

The fox is guarding the hen house
Wrong person in charge.

Fruitcake
Someone who is crazy.

Fruit of my loins
A baby that is the result of a man's semen.

FUBAR
An acronym used in past wars that stands for *Fucked Up Beyond All Recognition*, meaning it is as bad as it can get.

Fucked up
Drunk or stoned on drugs.
A situation is really bad, or

Fucking the dog
Being lazy.
Not getting work done.
Avoiding getting work done.

Fuck off
"Fuck" is one of the most used slang words and can
be the rudest.
Tell someone to go away.
Sit around and do nothing.

Fuck me
Have sex with me.
I give up.
Said in exasperation.

Fuck you
Said with vehemence, means you do not agree with
that person.
Angrily communicates that you really can't stand
that person.

Old fuddy duddy
A person who is old and doesn't want to be modern
or to change his ways.

Full of himself
Thinks he is the best or better than others.

Full of it
Liar.

Funny bone
Laughing.

Fussbudget
A person who is overly fussy.
A person who gets involved in other people's
personal business, but not in a helpful way, more like
an enabling and fomenting way.

G

(Big) galoot
A big guy.

On his game
Performing or thinking very well.

A gas
Fun.
Exciting.

Gave away the farm
Made a purchase or a pattern of purchases that is irresponsible.
Gave away ideas.
Gave away a mental platform of strength.
Gave away negotiating power.

Get a handle on
Figure out.

Get a life
Said to a person who worries about trivial things and the doings of others.
Don't concern yourself with others or their business.

Get back on the horse
Try again

Getting her hands dirty
Getting involved.
Lending a hand.

Get it off your chest
Talk about it.

Get it on
Have sex.

Get my ass handed to him
Beat up.

Get off
Have an orgasm

Get off his ass
Get up and do something instead of being lazy.

Get off on
Super enjoy something

Get out of Dodge
Leave.

Get serviced
Have sex.

Get some shuteye
Get some sleep

Get the scoop on
Learn about.

Don't get you
Don't understand what you are about, thinking, or doing.

Get off your can
Stop sitting and get up off your ass.

Get the dirt on him
Finding out the bad things about a person.

Get to the bottom of this
Find out.
Get the details on.

Get some
Get sex.

Get the skinny on
Get the full story, with details.

Get while the gettin's good
Leave while you can.

Get with the program
Learn.

Get your motor running
Grow increasingly energetic, often in anticipation of something.

Get your shit together
Get organized.

Gift of gab
Somebody who is good at talking.

A gimme
Easy.

Give it a whirl
Try.

Give it legs
Try.

Give no quarter
Don't give it a chance.

Green with envy
Extremely envious.

Don't give a shit/hoot
Don't care about it at all.

Give 'er hell
Go for it with zeal.

Give her an inch, she'll take a mile
Given a chance, she'll take advantage of.

Give it up
Get something from someone when they don't want to.
Return an item, especially in a situation where the person stole someone else's item.
Offers and gives sex.

Give him a piece of my mind
Tell him how you feel.

Gives me the willies
Makes me nervous.

Give up the ghost
Die.
Doesn't work anymore.
Broken.

Give up the goods
Tell.

Glad rags
Dress up clothes.

Go commando
Go without underwear.

Goes in the toilet
Fails.

Go for it
Undertake something with zeal.
Start it.

Go fly a kite
Leave me alone.
Go away.

Go getter
An achiever.
Hard worker.

Going in with your eyes wide open
Undertaking an endeavor that realistically will have
issues to face and obstacles to overcome, but not
resisting the endeavor because of it.

Going steady
Dating.

Golden goose
Something that gives a lot in return without much
effort.

Gold digger
Opportunist.

Gone belly up
Dead.
An endeavor has failed.

Gonna have your hide
Attack.
Get revenge.

Good answer
The answer the listener wants

Good job
Congratulations.
Sarcastically said that you did bad.

Good luck with that
Don't believe it's really going to happen.

Goody two shoes
Extremely straight-laced.

Googly-eyed
Enamored.

Goose is cooked
You're in trouble.
Someone found out and will punish you.

Got all your ducks in a row
Organized.

Got an axe to grind
Carrying a grudge.

Got bigger fish to fry
Have more important things to do.

Got cold feet
Scared.
Tentative.

Got it made
Successful.

Got snowed
Got fooled.

Go south
Fail.
Fall apart.

Go to town on
Beat up someone.

Got up on the wrong side of the bed
Grumpy.

Got your back
Help out.
Take care of.

Grass
Marijuana.

Green around the gills
Feeling like throwing up.

Grow thick skin
Not let things bother you.
Usually, if someone is saying something bad about you or to you, learn to ignore it.

Groovy
Cool.

Grow on you
A situation, person, or thing that you initially weren't feeling very favorable about, but after getting used to it, you think it's good.

Gun shy
Reluctant or scared.
Afraid of something.

Gung-ho
Really excited to do something.

Gussied up
Dressed up.

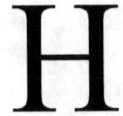

H

Half-assed
Doing partially well.
Doing a poor job.

Half in the bag
Partially or all drunk on alcohol

Hair of the dog that bit you
The dog that bit you is the voluminous amounts of alcohol drank a previous day.
The hair of the dog is having an alcoholic drink to help the person's hangover.

Hallway sex
When a married or cohabiting, unhappy couple passes each other in the hallway and says "fuck you" as they pass.

Ham-fisted (handed)
Awkward.

Hammered
Drunk

Hamstring it
Restricted.
Not up to speed.
Hindered.

Hands are tied
Nothing you can do about it.

Hand over fist
Often refers to money—that more money is
continually coming in.

Hang her out to dry
A person had been an ally to her, now faced with a
tough situation that could harm him in some way; he
lets her take the blame.
Betrays a person.

Got the hang of it
Learned how to do it.

Something to hang your hat on
An accomplishment that is your major endeavor.
An accomplishment that you are known for.
Something you believe in.

Hanky panky
Having sex or doing sexual foreplay

Happy as a clam
Happy.

Happy camper
Happy.

Hard to swallow
Not easily acceptable.

Happy go lucky
Happy.

Has a beef with
Have an issue with.

Has her eye on the ball
Watching.
Diligent.

Has his head up his ass
Oblivious.
Ignorant.

Has legs
Has a chance.
Has some value.

Has his head in the sand
Oblivious.
Ignoring.

Head's up
Watch out.

Hat in hand
Contrite.
Being apologetic.
Apologetic.

Has his head on backwards
Not thinking right thoughts.
His view or thinking is not correct.

Has his head on his shoulders
Wise.
Makes good decisions.

Haven't go squat
Have nothing.

Haven't the foggiest
Doesn't know anything.

I hear you
I'm listening.
I understand.
I agree.

Hauling ass
Going hard and fast at something whether it be
running or work or other endeavor.

Have another thing coming
Not what you expect.

Have it made
The situation is the best it can be.
Often means that a person has plenty of money,
perhaps a nice house and car, and profitably and
securely situated in a career, inheritance, or moneyed
marriage.
Have jack (shit)
Have nothing.

Have your cake and eat it too
Can't have everything your way.

Haywire
All amok or afoul.

Head case
Has a mental disorder.

Get your head out of your ass
Don't be oblivious.

Heads will roll
People will get fired from their jobs.
People will get in trouble or get disciplined.

Head screwed on straight
Clear thinking.
Good logical thinker.

Heavy, that's heavy, heavy, man
This is a holdover from the 60s and 70s, meaning deep intellectually.
Seeming deep because you're stoned on drugs.

Heinz 57
Like being like a dog that is a mutt.
From multiple racial origins.

Gone to hell
An endeavor or thing destroyed from its previous luster.

Hell bent on destruction
Determined.

(Went to) hell in a handbasket
Went bad.
Situation fell apart.

Hell on wheels
A person really determined to do something, whatever the consequences are.
A person who does bad or semi-bad things, but not necessarily illegal.

Hen pecked
Man who obeys his wife in everything.
Man who defers to his wife's wants.
A man who is considered less manly because he moves with his wife's wants.

Like herding cats
People or a situation that can't be made to flow in an orderly manner no matter how you try.

Hiding behind her skirts
Taking cover.
Cowardice.

Hinie
Bum or butt.

Hindsight is always 20/20
When looking back on a situation, things are clear.

Hit below the belt
Unfair attack.

Hit the road
Leave.

Hit it out of the park
A grand victory usually at work or sport endeavor.

Hit the ground running
Prepared to do something, so when it is time to start, he is ready to go right away.

Hit the bricks
Leave.

Hit the hay
Go to bed for the night.

Hit the head
Go to the bathroom

Hit the john
Go to the bathroom, with the room being called the john.

Hit the nail on the head
Got information or a situation extremely accurately.

Hit the pit
Go to bed for the night

Hit the sack
Go to bed for the night

Hit the wall
Can't go any further.
Hit the limit.

Hog out
Eat to excess.

Hold down the fort
Protect a situation.

Hold her own
Can keep up with others.

Holding his feet to the fire
Testing him to hold up to his words and actions.

Hold your tongue
Don't say anything.

Doesn't hold water
Doesn't stand up to scrutiny.

Has a hollow leg
Can drink a lot or eat a lot.

Holy cow/Holy crow/Holy mackerel
Wow!

Hokey
Not good.

Honey hole
For an endeavor, where the money is.
A woman's vagina.

Hoochie
Promiscuous person, usually referring to women.
Dresses and acts in an inviting, sexual way.

Horny
Amorous.
Sexually aroused.

On the hook
Owe money or other compensation for an activity.

Hooks into her
Attached, also as a situation.

Hook up
Have casual sex.

Hoodwinked
Faked out.
Deceived.

A real hoot
Having a good time.
A person is fun or funny.
A situation is fun or funny.

Hop to it
Start on something quickly.

Hoosgow
Jail.

Horking
Throwing up.

On the horn
Talking on the phone

A dark horse
A long shot that emerges when it was not thought to
win.

Beating a dead horse
Trying to revive a situation, but the situation is over and done, so it can't be revived no matter how hard you try.

From the horse's mouth
Heard from the original source rather than second or third hand or more.

(got) Hosed
Got taken advantage of.

Hot head
Angry person.

In the hot seat
As if the person was in a witness box in a courtroom. The person is very uncomfortable and feels like he is being attacked verbally.

Hot to trot
Horny.
Anxious to go.
Ready to go.

Hot under the collar
Angry.

How's it hangin'?
How's it going?

Eat a piece of humble pie
Becoming contrite.
Humbled.
Have to admit you are wrong and have to admit it.

Hummer
Giving a man oral sex while humming with your voice to produce a vibration on his penis.

Humping
Having sex

(Well) hung
Big penis.

Hungry
As in want badly.

Hung out to dry
Not offering any support.
Not helping out or coming to the aide of.
Being the one blamed even though others are also at fault.

Hunk
Very sexy man

Hunky dory
Doing well.
Feeling good.
In an agreeable mood.

I

I can take you
I can beat you up.

I'll let you live
I'll ignore that.

I'm easy
Sure.
Okay.
I agree.

Icing on the cake
Extra.

Idiot box
TV.

If it quacks like a duck, it must be a duck
If it looks like something, it probably is.

If it was a snake, it would have bit you
Not seeing the obvious.

If you live in a glass house, don't throw stones
Don't blame others when you have faults.

(get) In his face
Intimidate.

In deep weeds
In trouble.

In spades
Complete or solidly.

In the bag/got this one in the bag
Easy.
Done.
Finished.

In the dog house
In trouble.

In the game
In tune with the course.
With it.

In the klink
In jail.

In the loop
Kept informed.
Up to date on,

In a New York minute
Quick.

(Got the) inside track
Has the inside knowledge.

In the soup
In trouble.

In the tank
Drunk.
When something goes bad.

In the wind
Lost.
Disappeared.

Iron it out
Talk through.
Settled.
Smooth it over.

(Got) itchy palms
Money is coming or hoping it will.

It girl
Popular girl.

It's on me/her/him/you
My fault.

I've got this
I'll take care of it.

J

Don't have jack
Has nothing.

Jack of all trades and master of none
A person who can do many things, but hasn't pursued one avenue enough to be an expert in it.

Jacked up
A situation is bad.

Jack shit (ain't got)
Has nothing.

Jail bait
Underage female.

Jeepers Christmas
A euphemism for Jesus Christ said when something is exasperating.

Jerk off
Masturbating a man.
A man who is a jerk or idiot.

Jerk you around
Deceive.

(The) jig is up
The situation is now known. Often refers to
criminals involved in an activity and their actions are
now known and shut down.

Jing
Money.

Johnny on the spot
Someone there when needed.

Jump his bones
Have sex.

Got the jump on me
Beat me to it.

Jump the gun
Get ahead of yourself.
Start to run before they shoot the starting gun.

Jumping through hoops
Difficult task.
Getting past obstacles.

(His) junk
His testicles and penis.

It's a jungle out there
The terrain, the situation, the world can be
dangerous, such as said to a young adult going out
on their own.

Just for kicks
Just for fun for no particular reason.

Just peachy
Good.
Not so good (sarcastically).

TRISTAN JOHNSON

K

Kaibosh/kibosh
Put the stop on something.
Halt.

Keep my fingers crossed
Hope.
Hoping for the best.

Keep his head
Keep his wits about himself.
Keep cool under pressure.

Keeping you on your toes
As an example, in sprinting or ballet or other sport, the person has to be ready for action—literally on their toes.
A person has to be ready for whatever comes next.

Keep me on my toes
Keep sharp.
Pay attention.

Keep on truckin'
Keep going.

Keeps his cards close to his chest/vest
Secretive.

Keep your friends close and your enemies closer
Your friends you know are on your side so you don't
have to keep up closely with their thoughts and
actions regarding you, so you have to always know
what your enemies are doing to avoid being hurt.

Keep your stick on the ice
Pay attention.
Be ready.

Kept woman/man
A person financially supported while living with a
partner, and the first person does not earn an income.
This usually is used to apply to women.

Keester
Bum/button

Kick the bucket
Die.

Kick the can down the road
Instead of dealing with a situation now, it is put off
until later.
Instead of dealing with a situation, it is avoided by
giving the responsibility or blame to someone else.

Kick the tires
Try something out, but not necessarily with any
commitment.

Kicking it
Hanging out.

Kiss my ass
Fuck off.

Kill two birds with one stone
Accomplish two thing effort.
Solve two problems with one solution.

Kitty wampas
Crooked.
Out of alignment.

Knock on wood
A superstitious saying that by knocking on wood, the thing two people are discussing, won't happen.

Knock yourself out
Go ahead and do it.
Indifferent blessing or okay.
You can do that.

Knock your socks off
Really surprises you.
An experience that feels like a surprising, sudden change.
Really impresses you.

Knocking knees/boots
Having sexual intercourse in the missionary position,
so in theory, their knees would bang against each
other's.

In the know
Is aware of inside information or is involved in a
situation that is not widely known.
Knows a secret.

Koochie
Vagina.

L

Larger than life
Big
Important
Powerful

Lacksadaisical
Not done with proficiency.
Not done fully with attention to doing the details properly.
Doing something, but ignoring completing it properly.

Lady luck
Luck

Lame duck
They've been voted out of office, but are still holding the position until the new person is sworn in.

The last straw
Similar to drawing straws, where the person with the shortest straw must do something or win or lose something.
Where a person is entirely annoyed and exasperated with someone and that person does something wrong for the last time that the other person can stand.

Laughing my ass off
Laughing really hard.

Lay off
Stop.
Let up.

Laying a goose egg
Failing at an effort.
Losing.

Lech
Mooch.

Lead balloon
Bad idea or thought.

Leading her on
Implying or saying that he is interested in her
romantically when he really isn't because he just
wants sex.
Implying or saying that he is with her on a project or
endeavor when he really isn't.
Lying to make her believe he is on her side.

Leaving you high and dry
Abandon.

Left holding the bag
When a situation goes wrong, the other people
involved will quickly exit leaving you to take the
blame.

Let her hair down
Relax.
Open up.

Let it slide
Ignore.
Forgive it.

Let's let it percolate
Give the endeavor time to come to fruition. Often this means that the final outcome is guessed at but not necessarily fully known.

Let sleeping dogs lie
Leave the situation alone.
Don't antagonize.

Let the cat out of the bag
Telling the secrets.

Let the chips fall where they may
Let it go on.
Ignore it.

Let's boogie
Let's go.

Lick carpet
Perform oral sex on a woman.

Lickety split
Fast.
Right away.

Light a fire up his ass
Give the impetus to make someone do something
instead of being lazy.
Give someone the big motivation to do something.

A light bulb went off
An idea was suddenly thought of.
A concept, learning, or situation was suddenly
solved in one's mind.

Light in the loafers
Homosexual.
Gay man.

Lights are on, but nobody's home
Not very intelligent.

Light me up
Light my cigarette.

Light up my life
Make my life better and happier.

Like nobody's business
Done extremely well.

Lip service
Useless talk.
Talk about it but don't do anything.

Liquid courage
Booze.

Living hand to mouth
Whatever is earned is needed quite soon, so that the person can't get ahead financially.
Every month she is scraping to get by.

Living on the edge
Taking life on fully.
Undertaking endeavors with a dangerous bent to them.
Pushing boundaries.

Loaded for bear
Well prepared.

Lock, stock, and barrel
Everything.
All of it.

Long in the tooth
A person is old.

Lolly-gagging
Delaying.
Excessively slow.

It's a long story
Doesn't want to tell the story.

Look at it with fresh eyes
Come back to it later.

Looking down his nose at me
A person looking at another with disdain.
A person who thinks he better than someone else.

Looking down on others
As above

Look what the cat dragged in
A surprise.

Lose it
Lost your temper.
Lose control.

Lost his marbles
Went crazy.

Lost his shirt
Lost a lot of money, usually in a bad investment.

A lot on my plate
Have a lot to do.

Love handles
When someone is overweight, the phrase is used as a euphemism about the fat that accumulates about the waist.

No love lost
Two people don't like each other.

(On the) low down
Secretively.

M

Made in the shade
Has a situation that is ideal.

Madder than a wet hen
Really angry.

Made his own bed so he has to sleep in it
He created the situation, and now has to deal with it.

Made in the shade
Easy.

Make ends meet
Earn a living.
Having enough money.

Make hay while the sun shines
Do while you have the opportunity, while you have the chance.

Make some noise
Speak up.

Make the cut
Be good enough.
Be selected.

Makin' bacon
Fucking, as in sexual intercourse

Making a mountain out of a molehill
Making a big deal of something bigger than it
actually is.

Making pearls
This refers to how a woman's vagina looks like an
oyster. So, if a man and woman are having
intercourse on the beach, it refers to if sand gets in
her vagina, it would be like an oyster getting sand in
it, which makes a pearl.

Man about town
A debonair man who makes the round of better
social events.

A man's gotta do what a man's gotta do
If there is something that must be done, he does it
with no whining.

Man up
A man does what has to be done whether he likes it
or not.

Mary jane
Marijuana.

As mean as the day is long
Really mean.

Meat
Penis.

Meat head
Dummy
What Archie Bunker called his son-in-law in the TV series, *All in the Family*.

(Went) mental
Went crazy.

MILF
An acronym for "mother I'd like to fuck" that refers to sexy older women.

In her mind's eye
The way she sees it.

Mind your p's and q's
Be on your best behavior.
Pay attention.

Mixed bag
Good and bad.
Assortment.

Moment in the sun
His time to shine.
Crowning moment.

Monkey on my back
A habit or addiction that is really unwanted and really hard to get rid of.

More than one way to skin a cat
More than one way to do things.

All mucked up
Ruined.
Become in disarray.

Mucky muck
Important person.

Muddied the waters
Made unclear.
Added things to the situation that made the original concept or activity buried amongst the basic thing.

Music to my ears
A person has said something that the other person likes hearing because it is good or desired.

My hands are tied
Can't do anything about it.

N

Nailed it
Got it right.
Did something perfectly.
After trying hard or long, the person gets something right quickly, and the person is very happy about it.

Nailed her
Had sex with her

Namby pamby
Weak person.

Neat
Really pleasing, usually as in an idea or event.
Neatly tied up
A situation is finished in a satisfying way without loose ends to finish later.

Necking
Having a lengthy kissing session.

(That) neck of the woods
That part of town.

Hasn't got two nickels to rub/scrape together
Very poor.
Without the sustenance to survive.
Without financial prospects in the near or far future.

Nipping at our heels
Something catching up with you.
Pressing item.

Nip this thing in the bud
Take care of or address a situation.

No biggie
Not important.

No bones about it
Has no reservations.

No holds barred
There are no barriers to what you want to do.
To accomplish something, you will crash through
every barrier to your goal.

Nookie
Sex.

No pain, no gain
Have to work for something even when it seems
difficult.
No rest for the wicked
No rest.

No skin off my back/nose
Not an issue or concern.

Nose out of joint
Upset.

Nose to the grindstone
Working hard and diligently.

Not all it's cracked up to be
Not as good as it first appears.

Not feeling too hot
Feeling ill.

Not my cup of tea
Not what I like or prefer

Not out of the woods yet
Still more work to be done.

Not too shabby
Pretty good.

No worse for wear
Not damaged by circumstances.

Now you're cookin'
Things are going well.
On the right path.

Did a number on me
Did something bad to me.
Did something that later made me feel harmed
physically or emotionally.

Natural born sucker
A person who is innately easily duped.

(Go) nuclear
Get really mad.

Nuts
Crazy.

Nutty as a fruitcake
Crazy.

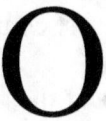

Oh, nuts
Darn.

Odd duck (duckie)
Unusual, unique or eccentric person.

Off base
Off target.
Wrong.

Off color joke
In appropriate such as racist or sexist.

Off on the right foot
At a good starting point with a new person.
Give a good first impression at first meeting a new person.

Off the cuff
Spontaneous.
Without much thought.
First thought.

Off the deep end
Jumped in.

Off the rails
Lost control.

Off the top of my head
First thought.

Off to the races
Quick start.

Old flame
Someone you used to be in love with.

Old lady/old man
A man's wife or girlfriend usually attributed to male (motorcycle) bikers as they refer to their women and vice versa.

On a losing streak
Things are going badly.

On her high horse
Looking down on others.

On his can
Fell down.

On his last legs
Dying.

On a short leash
Under control.
Restrained.

On the rag
Menstruating

On the tip of my tongue
When you know what you want to say, but you can't remember the word.

Once bitten, twice shy
Being tentative.

Once in a blue moon
Not very often.

On the ball
On target.

On the dole
On welfare or other government handouts

On the double
Go quickly.
Go now.

On the down low
Secretive.
Men having sex with men, but not talking about it.

On the fly
As you go.

On the fritz
Broken.

On the horn
On the phone or radio

On the lam
On the run.

On the level
Honest about a situation.
Telling the truth.

On the outside looking in
An outsider.

On the same page
Agree.

On the spot
Diligent.
Accurace.
Timely.

On the up and up
True.

On thin ice
Dangerous.

On the up and up
Truthful.

One trick pony
A person who does one thing of distinction or fame
and nothing else of notice follows.

On top of things
A situation is ordered and going smoothly. A person
has a situation under control.

Out cold
Sleeping hard.
Knocked out.

Not out of the woods yet
Not resolved.
Still in trouble.

Out on a limb
Taking a chance.
Testing the limits.

Out on his ear
Tossed out.
Forcibly removed.

Out there
Not normal.
Unusual.
Weird.

Out to lunch
Not very smart.

(Got me) Over a barrel
In a predicament

Overplay her hand
Said more than she can do.
Can't accomplish what she thought she could.

Over the hill
Old

Over the top
Extreme

Owly
Cranky.
Disagreeable.

Own up
Have enough character to announce your fault at
something and be willing to remedy the situation.

P

Packing heat
Carrying a gun

Pack it in
Stop it.
End it.

Padonkadonk
Rear end.

Paint the town red
Party hard.

Paint yourself into a corner
Get yourself into a situation you can't get out of.

(Didn't) pan out
Tried something and it didn't turn out as hoped.

Paper pusher
Person who works doing menial office work.

Paper tiger
Something that's made up to be bigger than it is.

Par for the course
What's expected.
Average.
Not surprising.

Partner in crime
Very close friend.
A person who is doing something with someone
else.

Party 'til you puke
Make the round of bars or at a house party drinking
to excess and doing activities that are excessive such
as doing drugs along with the alcohol.

Pass the buck
Blame someone else.
Not accept responsibility.

Pass the smell test
Not true.
Doesn't make sense.
Not believable.

Patsy
Someone who is targeted and blamed to be at fault
for something, usually by the perpetrator of the
action.

Pay Through the Nose
Pay a lot for something that shouldn't cost so much,
but you've gotta have it, such as a winter heat bill.

A peach
Something good or bad.

Peachy, peachy keen
Cool

Peanuts
Working for small amount.
Doesn't amount to much.

Pecker
Penis

Penny wise and pound foolish
Saves small amounts of money, then spends it all on big purchases that one does not necessarily need.

Pecker
Penis.

Pecker head
A low person who does stupid things unwittingly or willfully.
A person who is referred to as a penis because he is an idiot.

Pick up steam
Gain momentum.

Pie in the sky
Overreaching ideas or ideals that are not grounded in reality.

Piece of cake
Very easy to do with minimal effort.

Piece of tail
A person you want or did have sex with.

A real piece (of work) that one is
Difficult person.

Pie in the sky
Big dreams, but not necessarily fruitful.
Wishful thinking.

Pinch a loaf
Go for a poop

Piss ant
Insignificant.
Person who is insignificant.

Pissed off
Angry.

Piss tank
Drunkard.

Pissy
Cranky.

Plastered
Really, really drunk.

Plain jane
Normal and plain

Plays chicken
Seeing who will give in first.

Plays it close to the vest
Secretive.

Playing with fire
Engaging in an activity that has high potential for harm.

Play her along
Lead on.
Make her think something is not true.

Playing with the big boys now
Playing with superior people or people with power

Play the field
Not commit to anything or anyone.
Try different things.

Plum loco
Crazy.

Point fingers at
Accuse.

Poison the well
Make a situation go bad.
Injure.

Pokey
Jail

Pony up
Pay.

Poon
Vagina.

All pooped out
Exhausted, especially after doing an activity such as spring cleaning.

Poor as a church mouse
Religious people are credited with living an ascetic lifestyle, so a mouse living in a church would be poor also.

Porking
Having sex.

Haven't got a pot to piss in
Have no money at all and no assets worth much of anything.

Pressing flesh
Having sex.

Pretty penny
Expensive.

Pride goeth before a fall
A person with too much pride sets himself up for failure by not dealing with the situation as it is by thinking too much of himself.

Not with the program
Unaware of what's going on.
A little bit stupid, so the person doesn't understand what's going on.
Not doing things that the others want him to do.

The proof is in the pudding
The truth is obvious about something a person does.

Pull any punches
Hold back.
Refrain from.

Pulling her weight
Doing her share of the work.

Pulling the rug out from under him
Hindering.
Stopping.

Pull it off
Be able to do something that others would have not thought possible.
Sometimes a successful activity that is not necessarily very honest.

Pull the wool over her eyes
Deceive.

Pulled a boner
Did something really stupid.

Pulling my hair out
Upset.
Don't know what to do.

Pull the plug
Put an end to.

Pull strings
When a person asks for favors from influential people, usually from people who he has previously done favors.

Pull the plug on
An event or endeavor that gets shut down.

Punch drunk
A person who appears drunk with staggering or slurring speech as a result of being punched a lot—as in boxers.

Punk
A person, usually a man, who is a low, base person.
A person who cannot be respected or trusted with
anything.

Punked out on me
Quit.

Purple passion
Extremely passionate.
Often used to describe extreme dislike.

Push comes to shove
In the end it comes down to something.

Put words in her mouth
Misquote.

Puts her down
Says something about a person to others that is
negative or mean.
Says something to a person that is mean, almost to
the point of bullying.
Bullies a person.

Pushing the envelope
Pushing the limites.

Pushing 50
A person is almost 50 years old.

Push her buttons
Upset.

Pushing up the daisies
Dead and buried in the ground.

Put a sock in it
Shut up.

Put her foot down
Insist.
Demand.

Put him through the ringer
Give him a hard time and examine in great detail.
Question everything he says or does, as in
interrogate thoroughly. Think of an old ringer
washer and squeezing a person through the ringer.

Put that in your pipe and smoke it
There you have it.

Put his cards on the table
Be open, not deceptive.

Put the cart before the horse
Doing or thinking something before its natural
progression of one thing to the next in order.

Put the kaibosh on it
To stop something, squelch a person's plants, like a
veto, say "no."

Put the lid on
Hide.
To stop something.

Put this to bed
Get it done, resolved, or fixed.
Complete it.

(Feel) Put out
Feelings hurt.
Disrespected.
Ignored.

Put your best foot forward
Do your best.
Show your best.

Putz
Slow thinking person.

Q

Queer
Homosexual

Quit cold turkey
Quit something, like smoking, without an aid.

TRISTAN JOHNSON

R

Go down the rabbit hole
Get sidetracked.
Delving deeply into something and it turns out to be bigger than thought.

Raining cats and dogs
Raining heavily.

Raining on my parade
To spoil something.
Talking bad about.
Take the joy out of.

Raise the bar
Actively pursue doing more or better than before.
Creating an expectation of others that is higher or more forward than what is presently done.

Raising kane
Making a fuss.

Rake over the coals
Put someone through a tiring experience as a result of being questioned heavily.
Verbally accosted for an activity that the person did.

That's random
Something that is done or said that is bewilderingly unrelated to things previously said or done.

A rat
Tells on someone.

Rat race
Working for a living.

Rat (out) on him
Tell his secret.
Tell on him.

Rattle his cage
Deliberately cause a person to be confused or angry.

Read between the lines
Infer.

A real trooper
Hard worker.

Ream him out
Yell at.

Red Herring
Non-existent thing.

Red with anger
Very angry, usually that the person's face turns red from anger or if the person's face is not red, it is still described because the concept remains the same.

Riding the cotton pony
Having your period (menstruation)

Riding the red river
Having heterosexual intercourse when a woman is menstruating.

Ring my bell
A person who makes another interested sexually or amorously.

Rink rat
A kid who hangs around at ice rinks, sometimes playing pickup hockey and other times just hanging out.

Ripe for the picking
Ready.

Rip one
Fart.

Rip him a new asshole
Yell at him.

Ripping ass
Farting.

Rise to the occasion
Do what needs to be done.

(Get a) rise out of her
Get a reaction.

Robbing Peter to pay Paul
Borrowing from one to pay the other.

Rocks and sawdust in your head
Stupid.
Not learned.

Rock your world
A person has really great sex with another.
A person is really, suddenly in love.
Something is life-changing.

Rock your socks off
Creates an exhilarating feeling.
Surprises with an experience.
Less often used, but a band that puts on a super high-energy performance that exhilarates the audience.

Rolled on
Told on.
Let someone's secrets be known.

Rolling Sevens
Lucky.

Roll the streets up at night
Everything closes.

Learn the ropes
Learn what needs to be done based on past processes and practices.
Starting a job where you learn the company direction, practices, and culture.

A rose is but a rose
A situation or thing is exactly as it appears—nothing else.

Therein lies the rub
That's the underlying issue.

Rub elbows with
Hang out with.
Be around particular people, more likely important people, such as the upper class.

Rub her nose in it
Make someone feel bad about something.

Rub her the wrong way
Annoy.

Rub it in
Make someone feel bad about something.

Rub one out
A man masturbates.

Run for her money
A challenge.

Run it into the ground
Wear it out completely.

S

Sacred cow
Favorite cause.
Untouchable item.

(The) sandman is beating me to death
I'm really tired.

Save face
Avoid embarrassment.

Save it for a rainy day
Things in life are going well, but prepare for the worst by putting money aside for things that will not go well later
.

Saved my ass
Saved you from an adverse situation.

Sawing logs
Snoring loudly

Saw the writing on the wall
Saw it coming.
Knew it was coming.

Say what?
What did you say?

Scape goat
A person who gets blamed for something that they didn't do. Often it is the perpetrator who does the accusing.

Scare the dickens out of him
Really scared.

Scarf it down
Eat quickly and excessively.

Schlep over to
Go to.

Screw
Have sex.

Screwed
In trouble.
Things are not going well.

Screw her around
Cheat the person out of something.
Lied about a situation.
Cause a person to lose something by deceit.

Screwed him
This is basically the same as "Screw her around."
Had sex with a person, whether heterosexual or homosexual.
Often refers primarily to sexual intercourse involving a penis penetrating vaginally or anally.

Screw it
The heck with it.

Screw off
Not do what you are supposed to be doing.
Being lazy.
Go away.

Screw up
Make a mistake, but more often, to ruin a project or situation or relationship.

Screw you
Have sex with as in, "I want to screw you."
Angrily telling a person that you don't like them or don't agree with what they are saying.
I disagree with you and want you to go away.

See red
Angry.

See what's shakin'
Find out what's going on, usually to do with fun or is entertainment or a possible situation that could titillate.

Selling snake oil
Telling untruths.

Sell yourself short
Not taking enough credit.
Not believing in yourself.

Sent him packing
Told him to leave.

Her ship has sailed
It's too late.

Shagging
Fucking.

She's all that
She's good.

Shine a light on the situation
Make a situation known.

(Think his) shit don't stink
Arrogant.
Thinks a lot of himself.

Shit-faced
Really, really drunk.

The shit hits the fan
Get in trouble.

Shit hole
Bad place, such as a decrepit apartment

Shitting bricks
Really scared.

Shmoe
A loser.

Shoot me now
I'm done with it.
I want to quit.

Shoot the breeze
Talk with someone, usually about nothing very important.
Talk small talk.

Should talk to someone
See a therapist.

Shove it down his throat
Force it on him.

Shut me down
Don't let me do what I want to do.
Prohibited.
Put a stop to.

Skuzz bag
Unclean and avoided person.

Slam dunk
Easy.

Slap on the wrist
Easy or light punishment.

Sick
Means good.

Small potatoes
Unimportant.

Shrimp
Small person.

Shrinking violet
Shy.

Shut your face
Shut up.

Sitting on a gold mine
Have something that is prized and/or valuable.
A woman's vagina is worth gold to a man, so don't
squander it on lesser men.

Sitting pretty
In a good situation.

Skank/skanky
Nasty.
Dirty.
Unclean.

Skating on thin ice
Risky situation.

Skin in the game
Have a stake in.
Putting your name behind something.

No skin off my ass
No problem.
I can do it easily.

Slut
Promiscuous.
A woman who has many sexual partners for a night only. Increasingly it is used to describe men who are promiscuous.

Stick in my craw
Antagonizing.

Slipped a rufie
Gave a date rape or knock out drug without the other person knowing.

Slip through his fingers
Just missed an opportunity.
Had something good and unwisely let it go.

The shit flows downhill
This typically means in an organization with leaders that make a bad decision, and the results of the bad decision flows down the hierarchy of command to be a bad situation to everyone.
A decision is made and others in the organization have to deal with its consequences and try to fix it.

Shit for brains
Stupid

The shit hit the fan
Imagine shit being thrown at a fan and the fan spurts
it out all over the room. This idea is for a situation
that has blown up among people.
Really in trouble.

Skuzzball
Dirty person.
Unsavory person.

Small potatoes
Less important.

Snatch
Vagina.

Sold her out
Turned her in.
Told on.

Son of a gun
Unliked person.

Shooting blanks
A man's semen is not viable for insemination.

Shooting the breeze
Casual conversation.

Short a few marbles
Not that intelligent.
Missing some basic intelligence.

Shove it
Tell a person that you emphatically refuse their idea
or thought or activity, as in shove it up their ass.

Shove off
Go away.

Shoving it down her throat
Forcing a situation or idea on someone when that
person doesn't want to be forced.

Shut your trap
Told to stop talking

On a slippery slope
Risky situation.

Slow/quick on the draw
Sharp or not sharp intelligence.

Smart cookie
Smart person.

Smell a rat
Sense something is wrong.

Smoke and mirrors
Fake.
Deceptive.

(Where there's) smoke, there's fire
If there is evidence of something, most likely it is true.

Smoking gun
Evidence in a crime or other things.

Snafu
Acronym for "Situation Normal All Fucked Up"

Soft pedal
Speak lightly.
Soft sell.
Approach cautiously.

If it ain't something, it's something else
There are already negative things going on, then yet another negative or hard-to-deal with thing happens. Rarely get any peace from events to deal with that are not good.

Aw, snap
Darn.

Nothing to sneeze at
Worth admiring or valuing.

Snow job
Scam.

Something you can hang your hat on
Something you can count on or rely on.
For sure.
Known.

Went south
Fell apart.

Space cadet
Someone who is not very smart.
Off in her own world, and not quite grounded in
reality.

Spaghetti girl
Straight until wet, meaning a woman is heterosexual
when she is not horny, but is willing to have lesbian
sex when she is horny.

Spill his guts
Tell everything.

Spilling the beans
Telling.
Giving away secrets.

Spinning her wheels
Going nowhere.
Stuck.

Split
Left from somewhere.
Vagina.

Splitting hairs
Too much detail.
Going too deep.
Not a lot of difference.

Spot on
Accurate.
Right.
Correct.

Spread herself thin
Trying to do too many things and not giving each
one any focus.

Not a spring chicken anymore
Getting old.

Spun
Not mentally acute in a mental health kind of way.
Not that smart, but falls short of stupid.

Squared away
Corrected.
Fixed.

The squeaky wheel gets the most grease
The person who complains the loudest and/or the
most gets what they want faster than others.

(Don't know) squat
Don't know anything.

Acting squirrely
Acting goofy.

Got the squirts
Have diarrhea.

Stab in the dark
A guess.

Stand on your own two feet
Take care of yourself.
Independent.

Stand up guy
Dependable.
Honest.
Reliable.

Step up to the plate
A term from baseball about a person who goes to home plate ready to hit the ball.
Starting on something.
When others don't volunteer or accept responsibility, a stronger person assumes responsibility and authority.

On the straight and narrow
Honest
Less used, but to refer to overly religious people

Stick in the eye
Put a halt to.
Hurt.

Stick in the mud
The person is not any fun.
The person stodgy and not modern.
The person will not change with the times.

Stick to her guns
Persevere.

Sticky wicket
A problem.

Stir crazy
The ultimate in utter boredom.

Stoked
Excited about.

(Hasn't got) the stomach for it
Hasn't got the will to do it.

Stone-faced
Has no expression.

Stoner
Someone who does drugs.

Straight from the horse's mouth
The opposite of hearsay, meaning hearing the
testimony or story directly from the source person.

Stretch your dollar
Be financially economical.
Be frugal.

Strike while the iron is hot
Take advantage of the opportunity.
Act when the time is right.

No strings attached
No catches.

(Got) stood up
A person was going to meet you and didn't show.

Stuck up
A person who is not friendly in a haughty way.
A person who acts better than others, so refuses to be
acquainted with people she deems lesser than her.

Sucked in
Pulled into a situation.
Duped.

Suck it up
Quit whining and deal with it or do it.

Suck it up, princess/buttercup
A whining person who doesn't want to deal with or do a thing because she thinks she is too good for something.
Do it anyway.

You suck
You are not liked.
You don't do something well at all.

Sucks ass
Really bad.

Sucks (big fat) lemons
Too bad.

(So) sue me
So what.
I don't care.

(She/He can) suck the chrome off a bumper
The person can give an expert blow job.

Sugar coating
Makes it sound better than it is.

Swallow his pride
A person who doesn't want to be humble, who operates on ego and pride, but has to let go of pride and be humble, usually forced upon him by a situation or person.

Swan song
The last effort while waning into death or obscurity.

Sweep it under the rug
Pretend it doesn't exist.
Make the situation go away.

Sweet spot
The middle point that is the right place to be. For example, if you are buying a printer and need it for home use and anticipated amount of use. The $800 high-use printer would be too much, but the super cheap printer wouldn't accommodate your printing needs. So, a printer that falls in the middle will have landed on the sweet spot for a printer that does what is needed.

Sweet tooth
Likes sweet eats such as cakes, cookies, ice cream, or chocolate.

Swim with the fishes
In the water dead.

Switch hitter
Is bisexual.

T

Take a dump
Go for a poo.

Take a header
Have a rough fall.
Fall hard from a bicycle, snowboard, skate board,
motorcycle, etc.

Take a hike
Go away.

Take a leak
Go for a pee.

Take a pill/take your meds
Calm down.

Take a stab at
Try something.
Try something, but not necessarily whole-hearted.

Take a load off
Rest.
Relax.

Take a shine to
Like.

Take a stab at it
Try.

Take it in stride
Accepting.

Take it with a grain of salt
Believe, but not entirely.
Realize that it may not be inherently true because the
person has his own motives, so he may be not telling
all the truth, twisting it to his own ends, or
selectively omitting information or truth.

Takes the cake
Winner.
The best.

Take that to the bank
Can count on it.

Take the fall
Takes responsibility, that isn't necessarily yours to
assume responsibility.

(I can) Take you
I can fight you and win.
Smarter than you.
Better than you.

Take your eye off the ball
Not paying attention.

Takes him under her wing
Offers to teach a person and advance that person
who is worthy of that attention and favor.

Talking to Ralph on the big white telephone
Barfing in the toilet.

Talking out of school
Giving away secrets.

Take the bull by the horns
Take control of a situation without hesitation.
Takes control of a situation forcibly.

Talk turkey
Discuss details.

Talking out both sides of his mouth
Saying one thing, but is deceitful because his action
say another.
Saying two different things about the same thing.

Tanked
Drunk on alcohol.
It failed or crashed.

Has a tear on/on a tear
Going at it hard.
Determined.

Test the waters
See how amenable a situation is before committing
to it.

That blows
That's bad.

That's all she wrote
That's the end.

(She's) The shit
Really good.

Thick as thieves
Close together.
Working together.

My thing
His penis.

On thin ice
A person or an idea is wavering on yes or no.
If the person continues on a certain path, he may
metaphorically fall through the ice dead.

Has thin/thick skin
Tough or not.

The third rail
On a subway, the third rail in between the outer rails can kill you by electrocution. So, I heard this saying used about an issue that is the third rail for politicians, meaning it's an issue they are avoiding so it doesn't hurt or destroy their political career.

Thirsty
Zealous for an activity, goal, or outcome.

Three sheets to the wind
Really drunk.

Threw in a monkey wrench
Fouled it up.
Broke it.

Throw him for a loop
Upset it.

Throw in the towel
Quit.

Throw her hat in the ring
Volunteer for selection.
To run for election, as it is most commonly used.
Volunteer

Throwing good money after bad
Wasting money on a flawed premise or project.

Throwing her weight around
Bossing people around.
Using her clout or power to make others do the things she wants.

Through the ringer
Feeling beat up.

Throw him a bone
Do a favor or give in on something in hopes of getting something in return.

Throw him under the bus
Let someone else take the blame for something, usually a very bad outcome for the person under the bus.

Throw out the baby with the bath water
Don't throw out the whole thing just because some parts are bad.
Throw out the bad parts, but keep the good parts.

Thumbing his nose at
Dismissing.

Tighten his belt
Be more frugal.

Tight-lipped
Does not say much.
Will not reveal information about specific information.

Tight Wad
Has money but doesn't share it with others even
when the situation warrants it.

Tip of the iceberg
There's a lot more underneath.
Just the beginning.
A lot unseen.

Tits up
Dead.

He's toast
He is really tired.
In poor condition or in danger.
Warm and comfortable.

Took one for the team
Did their part.
Did more than their share.
Took some punishment for.

Tossed her cookies/lunch
Vomit.

Touch base
Check in with someone.

Touched
Mentally feeble.
Mentally ill.

It was touch and go
Could have gone either good or bad.

Tough call
Hard choice.

Tough go of it
Hard.

Tough nut to crack
A hard project.
A tough thing to do.
Hard to understand a person or task or problem.
Not easily understood.

Tough sledding
Hard going, like dragging a sled over rocks.

Towing the line
Behaving properly.
Saying what is expected.

Do the town
Go out for the evening and party a lot.

Train wreck
A real mess of a person or situation.

Tripping
Being very stoned on drugs, usually a hallucinatory drug like LSD, and experiencing a lot of hallucinations.

Try that on for size
Try it out.

Turn a blind eye to
Ignore.

Turn me on
Makes one feel sexually alive
A situation or activity makes you feel happy or interested.

Turn tricks
Prostitution.

Twat
Vagina.

Tweaker
A "meth head"—someone who does methamphetamines

Twist her arm
Try to convince.

Two cents worth
Your opinion or thought.

Two-faced
Deceitful.

Two peas in a pod
The same.

Two-timing
Dating two people at the same time.

U

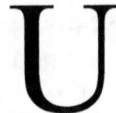

Under my belt
Experience.

Under the gun
Under pressure.

Under the radar
Secretive.

Under the table
Earning money that the IRS doesn't know about and you don't claim it on taxes.

Under water
In the negative, such as a check book being in the hole.

Under wraps
Keep something secret.

Under your nose
Something is done without you knowing, right under your awareness.

Undies in a bunch
Really upset feeling.
Unsure about what to do in an immediate situation.
Very worried.

Up for grabs
Open.
Could be anybody's.
Undecided.

Up in my face
Bothering.
Attacking.
Intimidating someone.

Up against the wall
Stuck.
No easy way out.

Up in the air
Undecided.
Could go either way.
Unknown.

Up the wazoo
Lots of.
Excessive amount.

Upper crust
Has high social standing, usually involving having a high net worth, usually with "old money," meaning that the family has been wealthy for generations, in contrast with those who are nouveau riche.

Upset the apple cart
Things or life are going along smoothly and peacefully. Then someone or an event throws things into disarray.

Up shit creek (without a paddle)
In trouble.
No easy way out.

Up your game
Get better at something.

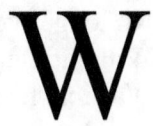

Wack job
Crazy.

Wait 'til it blows over
Wait until it passes.
Wait it out.

Waiting for the other shoe to drop
Expecting more bad news.

A walk in the park
Easily done using the least amount of effort.

Walk the talk
Take action, not just talk about it.

(Has a) wandering eye
Looking at other women who he is going to cheat
with.

A wash
The same.
Equal.

All washed up
No longer young and vibrant.
Without a future.
Was in a lucrative position or with a high ability, but no longer is. For example, a boxer who is past his prime and no longer wins the big fights would be called, "all washed up."

Wassup?
What are you doing?

Watch your back
Be careful.

Water under the bridge
A situation that has passed and does not affect a person anymore.

Water works
Crying.

Waxing the cane
Male masturbation.

Way to go
Saying to another person that they did great.

Wearing his heart on his sleeve
Very open at showing his emotions.

Wearing rose-colored glasses
Seeing a situation as ideal even though it is far from it.

Wears the pants in the family
In charge.

Wee wee
Penis.

Weiner
Penis.
Person who is dumb or unsavory in a way that is at the least, unsavory in a lascivious, sexually slimy way.

Well-heeled
Rich.

Went south
A project failed.

You're all wet
Lost.
Confused.
Mistaken.

Wet behind the ears
Brand new at something.
Not yet vetted.
Just born.

Whack job
A person who is really messed up in life, on drugs,
on a bad course in life.
A loser.

What am I? Chopped liver?
Not given any credit to.
Not noticing.

What gives?
What is this?
Expression of confusion or questioning.

When pigs fly
Never going to happen.

When it rains it pours
Things get worse.

When push comes to shove
At the final, when nothing else can be done. The
pressure is on and the situation is urgent, you have to
get done what has to be done.

When the chips are down
In a very serious, urgent or serious situation.
At a final, difficult, critical moment.

Whipper snapper
Young person.

White elephant
Non-existent.
Not a good idea.

Whole enchilada
The most, and often more, of a situation or thing.

Wild goose chase
Waste of time and effort.

In the wind
Got away from others.
Escaped.

Wind bag
Someone who talks incessantly.

Wild child
Usually refers to young women, who are willing to try anything, and usually do, sometimes to the detriment to their own safety.

Wishy washy
Indecisive

With a heavy heart
Feel sad.

(Not) With the course
Not paying attention.

(At my) wit's end
At my limit.

Wolf in sheep's clothing
Deceptive.
Hiding something worse than it appears.

Won't fly
Unacceptable.
Won't be accepted.

(It all) works out in the wash
It will even out.

Woopie ding
No big deal.
Nothing major.

Woopsie daisie
Oops.

Word
Agree with something.

Work like a dog
Work really hard and non-stop
Work him over
Question him really hard.

Work until her fingers bleed
Work past her limit of endurance.

Wound, Wound for Sound, All Wound Up, Tightly Wound
Can barely contain excitement.
Excited about something that will be happening.
Stoned on a manic feeling kind of drug.
Very anxious or worried so that it seems like the person will freak out at any moment.

Wrap my mind around it
Understand.

Wrapped around her little finger
Usually applied to women.
Will do anything for her.
Under her spell.

Wrecked
Drunk or stoned on drugs.

Saw the writing on the wall
Foresaw with observation that a certain event or situation would come to fruition, often meant that the situation would be very bad.

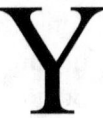

Yeah, man
This saying was heavily used in the 60s and 70s, as a relaxed, low-toned way of agreement.
A saying made popular in the Jamaican culture. It is a heavily used part of language that means acknowledgement during a conversation with an equivalent being "mm hmm" used to show a person you are listening. Or, it can mean a hearty agreement. It is often pronounced, "yah, mon."

Yippir
Yes.
Okay.

You are so dead
You're in trouble.

You dog
Unsavory character.

You scratch my back, I'll scratch yours
Trade off.
Help each other out.

You've got me there
I don't know.
Not sure what to do.
Not sure what to say.

Your ass is grass
In trouble.

Z

Zonked out
Sleeping hard, usually after a day of a lot of activity or illness.

Zoned out
Thinking in your own mind.
Not paying attention.